Low Carb:

90 Low Carb High Fat, Weight Loss Recipes For Healthy Living

Kris Tyson

I0423833

Table of Contents

Introduction   **10**

Chapter 1. Definition and Benefits a Low Carb Meal   **12**

Chapter 2. The Low-Carb Food List   **14**

Chapter 3. Low-Carb Breakfast Recipes   **17**

#1 Flaxseed Pancakes with Fresh Fruits   17

#2 Cremini Omelet with Spinach Filling   17

#3 Open-Faced Beef Burger on a Bed of Lettuce   18

#4 Omelet Muffinettes in Cheddar and Pecorino   19

#5 Morning Oatmeal Cookies   19

#6 Hominy, Bacon and Eggs Mornings   20

#7 Waffles with Cauli-Tomato and Chives   21

#8 Blueberry and Nectarine Granola Casserole   21

#9 Fried Cornmeal Crisps   23

#10 Crusted Cornmeal Couches   23

#11 Pancetta Rapa Frittatas   24

#12 Spanish Sausage Casserole   24

Chapter 4. Low-Carb Lunch Recipes   **26**

#13 Grilled Chicken with Salad Greens in Vinaigrette Dressing   26

#14 Spicy and Creamy Shrimp Brazilian Stew   28

#15 Zucchini Pasta in Basil and Pine Nuts Salad with Vinaigrette

Dressing   28

#16 Pork Frittata with Bacon and Butternut Squash   30

#17 Grilled Pork Chops in Mustard and Basil   30

#18 Pan-Fried Chicken and Tomato Salad   32

#19 Lamburger on Pita Bread   32

#21 Creamy Chicken Salad with Almonds and Berries   34

#22 Chunky Turkey with Rosemary and Garlic   35

#23 2-Cheese Mini Pepper Medley   36

#24 Garlic-Radish Tenderloin Tips   37

#25 Venison in Rosemary and Oregano Gyro   37

#26 Mexican Mango and Chicken Salad   38

Chapter 5. Low-Carb Dinner Recipes   **39**

#27 Chicken Breast Tomato-Zucchini Salad   39

#28 Salmon with Olives with Lettuce Side Salad   39

#29 Tuna, Black Olives, and Cherry Tomatoes Salad   41

#30 Pineapple Topped Teriyaki Beef Burger   42

#34 Cucumber, Tomato and Tofu salad   45

#35 Red Snapper Fillet with Olives and Feta Cheese   46

#36 Romaine Lettuce Salad with Anchovy Dressing   47

#39 Mexican-Inspired Cheesy Pumpkin Soup   49

#41 Creamy Oven-Roasted Onion and Tomato Soup   51

#43 Chicken Breast Tomato-Zucchini Salad 53

#45 Cranberry Salad in Watercress, Fennel with Balsamic Dressing 55

#46 Cheesy Garlic and Basil Pizza 56

#47 Turkey with Rosemary and Garlic 57

#48 Chicken Buffalo Crispy Fingers 57

#49 Turkey, Bacon and Spinach Scones **58**

#51 Tuna with Onions, Cabbage and Olives in White Wine Vinegar 59

#52 Stir-Fry Shrimp with Radish and Snow Peas 60

#53 Salmon with Parsnips, Broccoli and Dill 60

#55 Garlicky Ricotta Bacon and Baby Peppers 62

#56 Sautéed Asparagus, Capers and Pinto Beans 63

Chapter 6. Low-Carb Snack Recipes **64**

#57 Strawberry-Banana Flax seed Smoothie 64

#58 Banana-Carrot Smoothie 64

#59 Cherry-Almond Milk Smoothie 64

#60 Milky Low-Carb Papaya Smoothie 65

#61 Avocado Smoothie with Yogurt and Green Tea 66

#62 Berry Cinnamon Smoothie with Spinach and Chia 66

#63 Blueberry-Almond Smoothie 66

#64 Strawberry-Banana Yogurt Smoothie 67

#65 Orange, Soy Milk and Banana Smoothie 68

#66 Choco-Vanilla Peanut Butter Festive Latte　　　68

#67 Apple-Almond Yogurt Smoothie　　　68

#68 Peach-Banana Almond Milk Smoothie　　　69

#69 Apple-Avocado Milk Smoothie　　　70

#70 Banapple Vanilla Almond Smoothie　　　70

#71Vanilla-Apricot Smoothie　　　70

#72 Strawberry-Banana Flax seed Smoothie　　　70

#73 Banana-Carrot Smoothie　　　71

#74 Cherry-Chocolate Milk Smoothie　　　72

#75 Papaya Smoothie in Skim Milk and Honey　　　72

#76 Avocado Power Yogurt Smoothie with Green Tea　　　72

#77 Kale-Strawberry-Lime Smoothie　　　72

#78 Bok Choy Power Smoothie with Apples and Citrus　　　73

#79 Fruity Spinach and Ginger Smoothie　　　74

#80 Kale-Banana Smoothie with Coconut Flakes　　　74

#81 Chocolate Cookies in Soymilk　　　74

#82 Cinnamon Bar with Almonds and Apples　　　76

#83 Creamy Fruit Salad with Pecan Slivers　　　76

#84 Berry Nutty Fruit Salad　　　77

#85 Light Pistachio-Orange Fruit Salad　　　77

#86 Fruit Cocktail Cake with Butter Icing　　　78

#87 Mandarin Oranges and Pineapple Cake   79

#88 Strawberry with Almond-Vanilla Cream   79

#89 Bacon and Broccoli Egg Rollers   80

#90 Cinnamon-Vanilla Pumpkin Cuppycakes   82

Conclusion   **1**

CHECK OUT MY BOOK ON PALEO DIET: " A Beginner's Guide to the Paleo Diet: A Simple Start to Achieving Optimal Health and Weight Loss through the Original Human Diet + 35 FREE RECIPES"

Introduction

I want to thank and congratulate you for purchasing the book, *90 Days of Low Carbohydrate Diet Recipes"*

This book contains proven steps and strategies about the right kind of diet suitable for weight loss. According to medical journals, carbohydrates are components in modern day food that contain high levels of starch, and sugar.

The first chapter will introduce you to the world of carbohydrates. You will get to know what low carb is and how it benefits your body. For you to start eating healthy, you need to empty out or upgrade your pantry with the right food. Check out the list of suggested food items in chapter two.

Start your morning right with the low carbohydrate breakfast recipes. Chapter 3 has recipes that are designed to keep you full, satisfied and energetic. And since the gap between breakfast and lunch is crucial, fibrous components were included so you will not think about sinful sweets.

Take advantage of the hearty lunch you will learn in chapter 4. They are packed with delicious recipes you can even share with the entire family. Do keep in mind to eat heavy during the day to give your body time to digest the food. By having a heavy meal at night time, there are more chances of indigestion to occur. That is why you will learn more light meals for dinner in chapter 4. You can now plan your meals to include fish and vegetables that are easier to digest.

Should you get hungry in the middle of the night or you have an all-nighter at work, chapter 6 will show you how to prepare snacks that taste so good. Here's a hint: they have vegetables you can turn into a satisfying drink! Hurry now and let's begin the low carbohydrate eating transformation and see a big drop of weight in no time. Good luck and thank you for purchasing this book; hope you like it!

Chapter 1. Definition and Benefits a Low Carb Meal

Carbohydrates happen to be a core proponent of the American diet. However, if you are diabetic, too much carbs will cause your blood sugar to spike. Whole carbs make your body feel fuller for a longer period. Refined carbs make you hungry and want more food. The whole carbs you need to include in your meals are in the form of brown rice, beans, fruits, whole wheat pasta, vegetables and oats. The refined carbs are the sweet cereals, white bread, white rice, and concentrated fruits juices.

Remarkable Benefits of a Low Carb Diet

Low carbohydrates can help you lose weight, build muscles and keep you from feeling bloated. Here's why:

1. Food cravings are reduced.

   You are not missing out on nutrients when you eat low carb food. It is beneficial for your health, especially when you need to lose weight. Low carb food takes longer for you to feel hungry. Craving for sweets is reduced due to the low sugar content as well as the low salt content of the food you will eat.

2. Eggs are highly recommended to help build muscle mass.

   Eggs are high in protein that your body needs to convent fat into muscle. The energy that your body will store will help you maintain a more active and energetic lifestyle.

3. Water retention or bloating is reduced.

   The culprit to water retention is too much salty foods that you consume on a daily basis. Through a low carb diet, you lessen salt in your diet which will eventually allow you to prevent cardiovascular problems in the future. However, if you need to add salt to the food you will eat, choose Himalayan sea salt or kosher salt.

Chapter 2. The Low-Carb Food List

In the premise of your doctor's "good to go" signal, here is the list of foods that can complement this diet.

- Drinks
- Water
- Tea
- Caffeinated Coffee

- Dairy
- Whole milk yogurt
- Ricotta cheese
- Feta cheese
- Half-and-Half
- Cheddar cheese
- Parmesan cheese
- Eggs
- Cottage cheese
- Cheese
- Coconut Milk
- Cream cheese

- Bread, Beans and Nuts
- Saltine Crackers
- Oatmeal
- Granola/Bran
- Peanut Butter
- Whole-wheat bread
- Bagels
- Hummus

- Pistachios
- Walnuts
- Whole-wheat toasts
- Whole-wheat pasta

- **Fish and Meat (all)**

- **Fruits and Vegetables** (all but limit 1 serving/day for tropical fruits like pineapple, mangoes and watermelons)

- **Seasonings**
  - Beef broth
  - Chicken broth
  - Hot sauce
  - Catsup
  - Mayonnaise
  - Mustard
  - Balsamic vinegar
  - Apple cider vinegar
  - Red wine vinegar

- **Oil**
- **Canola**
- **Coconut oil**
- **Olive oil**
- **Others**
  - Cocoa powder
  - Flax seeds
  - Tempeh
  - Sesame seeds
  - Tofu
  - Stevia sugar substitute

Chapter 3. Low-Carb Breakfast Recipes

#1 Flaxseed Pancakes with Fresh Fruits

Ingredients

        3 tsp. coconut flour (substitute for baking powder)

2 tbsp. cane sugar

1 cup almond milk

1/2 cup water

1 tbsp. ground flax seeds

2 tbsp. apple cider vinegar

1/2 tsp. pure vanilla extract

3 tbsp. coconut oil

Agave nectar (topping)

Directions
- In a medium-sized bowl, add and mix all the ingredients.
- Heat a pan and pour the batter; cook for 4 minutes.
- Transfer the pancakes to a cooling wire; set aside for 3 minutes.
- Serve the pancakes with agave nectar.

#2 Cremini Omelet with Spinach Filling

Ingredients

1/2 tsp. turmeric

4 eggs

1 tbsp. arrowroot powder

2 tbsp. olive oil

Ingredients (for filling)

4 cups sliced Cremini white mushrooms

3 tbsp. fresh thyme (chopped)

2 tbsp. olive oil

2 cups fresh spinach leaves (chopped)

Directions

- In a food processor, add turmeric, eggs and olive oil; puree until smooth.
- Add arrowroot to the pureed mixture and blend.
- In a skillet, grease with little oil and cook egg mixture for 5 minutes before flipping.
- In a large pan, sauté the Cremini mushrooms, thyme and spinach with olive oil for 5 minutes.
- Stuff the spinach and Cremini mushrooms in the omelet.
- Serve on a plate and enjoy while hot.

#3 Open-Faced Beef Burger on a Bed of Lettuce

Ingredients

1 egg

1 shallot

1 lb. of ground beef (organic grass-fed)

3 cloves garlic

1/4 white onions (diced)

2 cups coconut aminos

White pepper (to taste)

Black pepper (to taste)

Directions

- Grind the onion, garlic and shallot with a mortar & pestle.
- Combine the mixture with the beef, egg and white and black pepper.
- In a skillet, sear the four mini patties with ghee.

- To make the sauce, simmer the coconut aminos and water for 2 minutes.
- On a plate, make a bed of lettuce and place the beef burgers on top.
- Add more flavor to the burgers by adding mustard or catsup.

#4 Omelet Muffinettes in Cheddar and Pecorino

Ingredients:
4 whole eggs
1 tsp. olive oil
1/4 cup Pecorino Romano (grated)
1 cup egg whites
1/4 cup cheddar cheese (grated)
4 cups broccoli florets
Kosher salt and pepper
Cooking spray

Directions:
- In a large pot, add water and steam the broccoli for 7 minutes.
- Set the broccolis aside in a pan, cut into small sizes and add kosher salt, pepper and olive oil.
- Meanwhile, beat the eggs, sargento cheese, pecorino Romano, pepper, kosher salt and egg whites in a bowl.
- Pour the egg mixture muffin pan pre-sprayed with cooking spray.
- Bake omelet for 20 minutes at 350 degrees F.
- Transfer the omelet muffinetes onto a plate and top with extra pecorino romano.

#5 Morning Oatmeal Cookies

Ingredients
1/2 cup cane sugar
1/2 cup low-fat butter

1 kiwi, puree
2 cups almond milk
2 1/4 cups chickpea flour
2 tsp. vanilla extract
1 tsp. baking soda substitute*
1 cup oat cereal
2 cups oatmeal

Directions

- To make the baking soda substitute* you need 4 tbsp. water, 1 tbsp. ground flax seed, and 1 tbsp. agar agar powder.
- All you have to do is simmer 3 tbsp. water and ground flax seed for 3 minutes in a pan.
- In a bowl, dissolve the agar agar powder with one tbsp. water; whip until frothy.
- Place in the refrigerator's chiller for 30 minutes. Serve on a plate and enjoy!

#6 Hominy, Bacon and Eggs Mornings

Ingredients

1 can hominy (maize kernels)
4 eggs
¼ pound sliced bacon
¼ cup chopped onion
1/4 tsp. pepper

Directions

- In a skillet, add onions and bacon; cook until the bacon is crispy and onions are tender.
- Stir in pepper, beaten eggs and hominy; cook until eggs are set.

#7 Waffles with Cauli-Tomato and Chives

Ingredients

2 eggs

1 tbsp. sun-dried tomatoes

1 tbsp. chives

1 cup cauliflower

1/3 cup parmesan cheese

1/2 tsp. pepper

1 tsp. onion powder

1 cup mozzarella cheese

1 tsp. garlic powder

Directions:

- In a large bowl, add the beaten eggs; combine with sun-dried tomatoes, chives, cauliflower, parmesan cheese and mozzarella cheese.
- Add the onion and garlic powder.
- Use a waffle maker to place the eggs and vegetable batter; add a pinch of pepper to taste.
- Cook the omelet waffle for 6 minutes.
- Once done, transfer onto a plate and serve.

#8 Blueberry and Nectarine Granola Casserole

Ingredients
2 tbsp. orange liqueur
1 cup almond Fruit granola
1/2 cup fresh blueberries
4 medium nectarines
2 tbsp. cane sugar

Directions

- Preheat your oven to 450 degrees F.
- In a medium bowl, mix together the blueberries, orange liqueur and nectarines.
- In a casserole, add in the sliced fruits, add the cane sugar and pop the casserole in the oven for 8 minutes until the fruits are tender.
- Serve on a plate then enjoy the sweet and succulent fruits on a casserole treat.

#9 Fried Cornmeal Crisps

Ingredients
½ cup fat-free milk
1 cup water
1/4 cup oil
1 tbsp. baking powder
2 cups yellow cornmeal
Confectioner's sugar (for dusting)

Directions
- All you have to do is mix ¼ cup of oil and add the milk, water, baking powder and cornmeal in a bowl.
- Pour the batter in a hot iron skillet and cook on low heat for 15 minutes.
- Once the cornmeal crisps are done, dust confectioner's sugar on top and serve on a plate.

#10 Crusted Cornmeal Couches

Ingredients
2 eggs
4 cups corn meal
2 tsp. baking powder
1/2 cup vegetable oil
1 tbsp. unsalted butter

Directions
- Begin by heating the oil in a pan.
- In a small bowl, moisten the cornmeal with warm water then add eggs and baking powder.
- Pour the cornmeal mixture into the hot vegetable oil.
- Cover the pan and wait until the crust is set.
- Remove from the pan and serve with a glass of soy milk on the side.

#11 Pancetta Rapa Frittatas

Ingredients

6 strips of bacon (reserve drippings for cooking)

1 lb. Turnip

8 pieces of minced baby bellas

2 leeks (washed and sliced)

1 tsp. nutmeg

1 tsp. kosher salt

1 can of coconut milk

4 pieces of Scallions (washed and sliced)

1/4 tsp. ground black pepper

Directions:

- Cook the bacon strips in a non-stick pan then set aside; reserve the bacon fat for frying.
- Shred the turnips and transfer them in a mixing bowl.
- Add the bacon fat and combine it with black pepper, nutmeg, kosher salt, leeks, and coconut milk.
- Transfer the turnip mixture to a 2 quart dish.
- Top the turnip mixture with bacon, baby bellas and scallions.
- Bake for 1 hour at 350 degrees F and serve hot.

#12 Spanish Sausage Casserole

Ingredients

1/2 piece green bell pepper (chopped)

Ground black pepper (to taste)

Freshly minced dill (for garnishing)

Oregano (dried)

10 organic eggs (medium)

1 lb. chorizo

2 cups onions (chopped)

Directions

- While cooking the chorizo in a skillet over medium heat.
- In a large bowl, whisk eggs and add the onion, black pepper, green pepper, and oregano.
- Add the chorizo to egg mixture and gently combine together.
- Pour the egg mixture into a baking dish and sprinkle freshly minced dill on top.
- Bake for 30 minutes at 350 degrees F.
- Serve on individual plates and enjoy with a cup of black coffee.

Chapter 4. Low-Carb Lunch Recipes

#13 Grilled Chicken with Salad Greens in Vinaigrette Dressing

Ingredients
1/2 tsp. dried thyme
4 pieces chicken breast halves
1/4 cup cider vinegar
1 and 1/4 tsp. onion powder
1 tbsp. water
4 tbsp. salad oil
1 medium carrot
1/4 tsp. dry mustard
1 small red sweet pepper
1/2 tsp. black pepper
1/4 tsp. garlic powder
1 green onion
6 cups mixed salad greens

Directions
- Set your grill temperature to 170 degrees F.
- Combine the onion powder, salad oil, and pepper.
- Brush the oil mixture on the chicken and grill for 15 minutes until cooked through.
- Combine the mixed salad greens, green onion, red sweet pepper, and carrots in a large salad bowl.
- Add the chicken and pour the dressing before serving.

Dressing Ingredients
½ cup salad oil
1 tbsp. cider vinegar
1 tsp. garlic powder

1 tbsp. mustard
1 tbsp. water
1 tsp. onion powder
1 tsp. dried thyme

Dressing Directions
- In a glass jar, combine the salad oil, cider vinegar, mustard, water, dried thyme, onion powder, and garlic powder.
- Shake the ingredients and drizzle on the chicken.

#14 Spicy and Creamy Shrimp Brazilian Stew

Ingredients
¼ cup red pepper (roasted)
¼ cup fresh cilantro
1 clove garlic
1½ lbs. shrimp
2 tbsp. lime juice (freshly squeezed)
¼ cup olive oil
1 can diced tomato
2 tbsp. hot sauce
1 cup coconut milk
¼ cup onion
Kosher salt and pepper (to taste)
6 bowls of Risotto (optional)

Directions
- In a pan, add olive oil and sauté the chopped onions, red peppers and garlic.
- Add in the cilantro, shrimp, tomatoes, hot sauce and coconut milk.
- Heat to a rolling boil and add kosher salt, pepper and lime juice to taste.
- Add a bowl of risotto and serve stew in ceramic bowls; garnish with extra cilantro.

#15 Zucchini Pasta in Basil and Pine Nuts Salad with Vinaigrette Dressing

Ingredients
1 package Parmesan cheese
1 package of zucchini pasta

1/2 cup pine nuts

1/3 cup red wine vinegar

1 tsp. ground pepper

1 garlic clove

1 tsp. mustard

1 cup fresh basil

3/4 cup olive oil

Grape tomatoes (for garnishing)

Mixed salad greens (for garnishing)

Yellow tomatoes (for garnishing)

Directions

- In a medium pot, add water and boil the small pasta shells until al dente.
- To prepare the dressing, whisk the vinegar, oil and pepper in a medium bowl.
- Once the pasta is cooked, add the vinaigrette dressing over it and add the basil, pine nuts and cheese.
- In a plate, add grape tomatoes, mixed salad greens and yellow tomatoes.
- Toss all the salad ingredients and top with grated Parmesan cheese.
- Serve in individual plates, garnish with grape tomatoes, yellow tomatoes and mixed salad greens.

#16 Pork Frittata with Bacon and Butternut Squash

Ingredients
10 eggs
1 lb. ground pork
1/4 tsp. ground mace
3 cups butternut squash (chopped)
4 thick slices bacon (chopped)
2 sprigs of thyme
1 tbsp. fresh sage (chopped)

Directions

- In a pan, cook the bacon to a crisp for 5 minutes.
- Layer in a pan the ground mace, thyme, ground pork, and sage.
- Add the butternut squash, eggs and thyme; cook on low for 2 hours; remove pan and serve frittata.
- Garnish with the bacon strips and enjoy!

#17 Grilled Pork Chops in Mustard and Basil

Ingredients

4 pork chops

1/2 cup mustard

1/4 cup olive oil

1 small diced shallot

1 tsp. ground cardamom

3 tbsp. raspberry vinegar

Ground pepper (to taste)

1/4 cup finely shredded basil (reserve one leaf for garnishing)

Directions

- On a plate, allow the chops to sit at room temperature for about an hour.
- Sprinkle each chop side with pepper; spread the mustard.
- In a medium sized bowl, add and combine all the ingredients; sprinkle pepper to taste.
- Grill the chops for 6 minutes on each side at 375 degrees F.
- Flip the chops when grill marks have already appeared; baste the chops with mustard.
- Serve the grilled chops on a plate and garnish with basil.

#18 Pan-Fried Chicken and Tomato Salad

Ingredients
½ lb. chicken breasts
1 and 1/2 tbsp. dried lime
1 tbsp. advieh seasoning (store-bought)
1/2 tsp. freshly ground black pepper
1 tbsp. oil

Directions

- In a grinder, grind the Persian dried lime until it turns to powder.
- In a small bowl, mix the Persian advieh seasoning, and pepper
- Cut each chicken in half and rub the advieh seasoning mixture.
- In a skillet, pour oil and sauté the chicken until they turn golden brown.
- Remove from the skillet and drain the chicken on paper towels.
- Serve the chicken with tomato and feta salad on the side.
- Layer the meat on top of the warmed pita bread and serve.

#19 Lamburger on Pita Bread

Ingredients

1/2 lb. lean ground lamb

2 cloves garlic

1 slice pita bread

1/2 onion

1/2 lb. lean ground beef

1/2 tsp. ground allspice

¼ ground cumin

1/2 tsp. ground coriander

1/2 tsp. ground black pepper

1/2 tsp. advieh seasoning

Directions

- Preheat a grill and grease the grate with oil.
- In a large bowl, combine ground land, garlic, onion, ground beef and bread crumbs.
- Season it with allspice, coriander, pepper and advieh seasoning.
- Knead the mixture and shape into 4 thin patties.
- Grill the patties for 7 minutes on each side; once done, transfer to a plate and serve.

#20 Beef Sirloin Kebab with Onions and Plantain

Ingredients
1 plantain
1 tbsp. Taco seasoning
1 tbsp. cooking oil
1 large beef sirloin steak (cut into cubes)
1 medium red onion
2 tbsp. red wine vinegar

Directions

- Preheat your grill and spray cooking oil.
- Remove excess fat from the sirloin steak.
- In a small bowl, mix red wine, vinegar, taco seasoning, oil and steak cubes.
- Toss the ingredients together to coat the meat and set aside.
- Take the skewers and thread the chunks of meat, onions and plantain.
- Brush the kebabs with olive oil and grill until the meat and vegetables are cooked.
- When you achieved the grill marks on the kebabs; serve right away.

#21 Creamy Chicken Salad with Almonds and Berries

Ingredients

4 tbsp. cream cheese

1 cup mayonnaise

2 tsp. curry powder

6 cups cooked chicken

2/3 cup dried cranberries

1 cup almonds

Direction

- In a large bowl, add the cream cheese, and curry powder.
- Whisk the ingredients until the cheese is fully coated by curry then mix the cranberries and chicken.
- Transfer the mixture on a plastic covered round cake pan and refrigerate overnight.
- The following day, remove the plastic cover and invert the cake pan on a plate.
- Toss the salad and garnish with chopped almonds and cranberries on top.

#22 Chunky Turkey with Rosemary and Garlic

Ingredients

3 cloves garlic

2 lb. turkey chunks (thinly sliced)

1/4 cup fresh lemon juice

1 tbsp. black peppercorns

2 tbsp. fresh rosemary

2 tbsp. olive oil

Directions
- Preheat your grill and grease the pan with cooking spray.
- In a medium-sized bowl, add the garlic, turkey chunks, lemon juice, peppercorns and rosemary; refrigerate for 1 hour.
- Remove the turkey from marinade.
- In a pan, cook the turkey for about 4 minutes; add the remaining lemon juice.
- Serve on a plate and garnish with rosemary leaves.

#23 2-Cheese Mini Pepper Medley

Ingredients
6 ounces soft goat cheese
1 tsp. garlic powder
15 sweet mini peppers
15 bacon strips
1/2 cup skim ricotta cheese
Pepper (to taste)

Directions
- Set oven to broil and line a baking sheet with foil; set aside.
- In a small bowl, add the ricotta, seasonings and goat cheese.
- Pipe in the cheese mixture into the halved peppers; wrap in bacon.
- Broil the arranged peppers for about 56 minutes until it turns nicely brown before serving on a plate.

#24 Garlic-Radish Tenderloin Tips

Ingredients

1 lb. tenderloin steak
Ground black pepper (to taste)
2 pieces radish
1 and ½ tbsp. oil
2 cloves garlic
2 tbsp. sake
Scallions (for garnishing)

Directions

- In a bowl, add the grated radish, scallions and garlic.
- On a chopping board, trim off excess fat from the tenderloin tips; season it with pepper.
- In a frying pan, add oil and sauté the garlic until lightly brown.
- Transfer the garlic on paper towels to drain excess oil; retain garlic oil in the pan.
- Cook the steak in the pan until it turns brown; flip to continue cooking the other side.
- Pour sake and shake pan to distribute evenly.
- Place the tenderloin tips on a plate; garnish with grated radish, crunchy garlic and scallions.

#25 Venison in Rosemary and Oregano Gyro

Ingredients

3 lbs. venison
1 package pita bread
2 tsp. ground dried rosemary
2 tbsp. olive oil
2 tsp. dried marjoram
Pepper (for seasoning)
1 tbsp. minced garlic

1 and 1/2 tbsp. ground cumin
1 tbsp. red wine vinegar
1 tbsp. dried oregano

Directions

- In a large ceramic bowl, add the cumin, marjoram, garlic, rosemary, red wine vinegar, venison strips, oregano, and pepper; toss to coat the meat.
- Cover the ceramic bowl and refrigerate the marinade for about 2 hours.
- Cook the venison strips in a large skillet for about 8 minutes until golden brown.

#26 Mexican Mango and Chicken Salad

Ingredients:
1 head of romaine lettuce
2 cups chicken enchilada (store-bought)
1 mango
½ avocado
Pepper and kosher salt (to taste)

Directions:

- On a plate, add shredded romaine lettuce and top with heated chicken enchilada.
- Slice the avocado and mangos into wedges; add them on top of the chicken.
- Sprinkle pepper and kosher salt to taste and serve without any dressing since it already tastes perfectly awesome!

Chapter 5. Low-Carb Dinner Recipes

#27 Chicken Breast Tomato-Zucchini Salad

Ingredients

2 chicken breasts

2 tbsp. tomato sauce

1/4 cup black olives

1/2 tsp. oregano leaves

½ cup green bell pepper

1 tbsp. light butter

½ cup yellow bell pepper

2 medium zucchini

½ cup red bell pepper

Directions
- Preheat your oven to 250 degrees F.
- In a bowl, add the chicken breast and sprinkle it with salt.
- In a foil wrap, add the zucchini slices and assorted bell peppers.
- Top the vegetable mixture with the chicken, oregano, butter, tomato sauce and olives.
- Wrap the foil and bake for 30 minutes.
- Unwrap the foil and serve immediately.

#28 Salmon with Olives with Lettuce Side Salad

Ingredients

1/2 cup black olives
1 can of salmon (in water)
2 cups fresh curly parsley
1/2 red onion
1 head romaine lettuce
2 tbsp. white wine vinegar
Pepper (to taste)
1 egg
1/4 cup of olive oil

Directions
- In a salad bowl, add white wine, vinegar, egg, and pepper; whisk to emulsify.
- Add the rest of the ingredients and toss to combine.
- Serve right away or keep refrigerated before serving.

#29 Tuna, Black Olives, and Cherry Tomatoes Salad

Ingredients
6 large lettuce leaves
2 cups trimmed green beans
2 cans tuna (packed in water)
4 cups romaine lettuce
4 anchovy fillets
1 and ¼ lb. small red potatoes
6 large pitted black olives, sliced
12 cherry tomatoes
2 tbsp. lemon juice
1 large egg (hard-boiled)
2 tbsp. red wine vinegar
1 tbsp. olive oil
¼ tsp. black pepper

Directions
- In a large saucepan, bring water to a boil and add green beans and potatoes.
- Remove the green beans after 6 minutes, but continue boiling the potatoes for about 12 minutes.
- Meanwhile, arrange a bed of lettuce leaves on a plate and place the cherry tomatoes, eggs, green beans and tuna.
- Sprinkle anchovy fillets and olives on top.
- In a small bowl, add the olive oil, black pepper, red wine vinegar, and lemon juice; stir to combine; drizzle on top of the salad.

#30 Pineapple Topped Teriyaki Beef Burger

Ingredients

1 can of pineapple rings

1 soy burger

8 slices cheddar cheese (fat-free)

8 hamburger buns

1 head of lettuce

1 tomato

1 bottle of mayonnaise (fat-free)

1 bottle of thick teriyaki marinade

Directions

- In a pan, coat with cooking spray and add a pineapple ring; cook until caramelized; set aside.
- Microwave the soy burger and place on the opened bun.
- Top the burger with teriyaki marinade, add cheese; microwave for 30 seconds.
- Once the cheese melts, add the pineapple ring on top and cover the soy burger.
- Garnish with a slice of tomato and a romaine lettuce leaf; serve immediately and enjoy!

#31 Sirloins and Mixed Greens Salad

Ingredients

8 cups mixed salad greens

1 recipe buttermilk dressing *

1 medium yellow sweet pepper

1/4 cup fresh basil

8 ounces beef sirloin steak

2 medium carrots

1 cup cherry tomatoes

Cooking spray

Directions
- Grease a large skillet with oil and add the meat and basil.
- Cook the meat for about 3 minutes then remove the skillet from the heat.
- On a large serving plate, place the carrots, salad green, sweet pepper and tomatoes.
- Trim excess fat from the meat and slice them into thin strips.
- Serve the sirloin steak salad, pour buttermilk ranch dressing and garnish with sliced tomatoes.

Ingredients for the Low Calorie Buttermilk Dressing*
2 tbsp. white-wine vinegar
1/4 cup mayonnaise reduced-fat
1/2 cup buttermilk
1/2 tsp. garlic (granulated)
1/3 cup chopped fresh herbs (tarragon, chives, basil)
1/2 tsp. pepper

Directions
- In a medium-sized bowl, combine mayonnaise, buttermilk, white wine vinegar, and pepper.
- Stir the ingredients until they become smooth.

#32 Pork Tenderloins with Mashed Cauliflower

Ingredients
1 cup chicken broth
2 pork tenderloins (trimmed fat)
1 can of organic mushrooms
2 tbsp. oregano
1 tbsp. basil
1 tbsp. garlic powder
2 bay leaves
1 large can organic tomatoes (diced)

Directions
- In a crockpot, add pork tenderloin, diced tomatoes, mushrooms and spices.
- Lastly, pour the chicken broth and cook for 8 hours on low heat.
- Once the tenderloin is cooked, transfer to a plate and garnish with mushrooms.

Ingredients for the Mashed Cauliflower
2 tbsp. Butter
1 head Cauliflower

Directions
- Steam cauliflower, butter and pepper for 30 minutes and puree in blender.
- Serve the mashed cauliflower and pork.

#33 Plantains and Onions Skewered in Pork Cubes

Ingredients
2 ripe plantains
1 tbsp. Taco seasoning
1 tbsp. cooking oil
12 ounces pork (cubed)
1 medium red onion

2 tbsp. red wine vinegar

Directions
- Preheat your grill and spray cooking oil.
- Remove excess fat from the sirloin steak.
- In a small bowl, mix red wine, vinegar, taco seasoning, oil and pork.
- Toss the ingredients together; set aside for 30 minutes for the pork to marinade.
- Afterwards, take the skewers and thread the chunks of pork, onions and plantain.
- Brush the kebabs with olive oil and grill until the pork and vegetables are cooked.
- When you achieved the grill marks on the kebabs, serve them immediately with a side dish of yogurt dip.

Ingredients for the Yogurt Dip
1/2 cup plain yogurt
1/3 cup feta cheese
1 tsp. lemon juice
1 garlic clove
1/2 tsp. pepper
1/2 tsp. hot pepper flakes
1/2 tsp. dried mint

Directions
- In a food processor, add in the crumbled feta cheese, pepper, dried mint, lemon juice, plain yogurt, garlic clove, and pepper flakes.
- Set the processor to a pulse and blend the ingredients to achieve a smooth dip.
- Transfer the yogurt dip in a small bowl and serve.

#34 Cucumber, Tomato and Tofu salad

Ingredients
Handful chopped fresh basil
1 tin kidney bean
        Freshly ground black pepper (to taste)
1 cucumber

1 tomato
1/2 red onion
100g firm tofu
4 tbsp. salad dressing of choice
Romano cheese (for topping)

Directions

- In a large bowl, combine the cucumber, red onion, kidney beans, tofu, tomato and basil. Toss with balsamic dressing, season with pepper.
- Serve on plate and enjoy with fresh shavings of Romano cheese.

#35 Red Snapper Fillet with Olives and Feta Cheese

Ingredients
¾ pound red snapper fillets
2 tbsp. black olives
2 tbsp. olive oil
2 tbsp. low-fat feta cheese (crumbled)
½ cup carrots
1 large tomato
1 clove garlic
½ cup dry white wine
1 medium onion
½ cup red pepper

Directions

- In a medium-sized skillet, sauté the carrots, red pepper, onions and garlic with olive oil; cook for 10 minutes.
- Add white wine and bring to a boil.
- Place the fish fillets in the same skillet and cook for about 5 minutes; add the olives and tomatoes.

- Cook the fillets for about 3 minutes top with cheese.
- Transfer to a serving plate; garnish with the skillet's juices and cooked vegetable.
- Serve with ½ cup of cooked brown rice.

#36 Romaine Lettuce Salad with Anchovy Dressing

Ingredients

8 cups small romaine lettuce leaves

1 cup whole grain bread (cubed)

3 tbsp. chicken broth (reduced-sodium)

1 tbsp. olive oil (extra-virgin)

1 tsp. cider vinegar

1 tsp. parsley (chopped)

1 small garlic clove

1 tsp. anchovy paste

2 tbsp. Parmesan cheese (grated)

1 tbsp. mayonnaise (reduced-fat)

1 tsp. Dijon mustard

A pinch of black pepper

Directions
- To make the croutons, preheat your oven to 350 degrees F.
- In a small baking bowl, put the bread cubes and bake in the oven for 10 minutes.
- In a medium-size bowl, add the pre-mashed garlic, 1 tablespoon of parmesan cheese, mayonnaise, oil, vinegar, parsley, pepper, anchovy paste and garlic paste.
- In a bowl, add the croutons and romaine lettuce; toss with the dressing.
- Top with parmesan cheese and serve into smaller plates.

#37 Roasted Crusted Lamb in Merlot

Ingredients

3 tbsp. dried cranberries
1 cup merlot
1/2 tsp. nutmeg
2 cloves garlic
2 1lb. lamb rib roast
1 tbsp. fresh rosemary
3 tbsp. olive oil
1 tbsp. butter
1 tbsp. fresh rosemary
2 cups soft bread crumbs
1/2 tsp. black pepper
1 tbsp. dried lavender

Directions

- Preheat your oven to 450 degrees F.
- On a chopping board, slice off the membrane and fat layers of lamb.
- Once done, prepare the marinade by placing the lamb roast, clove garlic, merlot and nutmeg in a zip-lock bag and place it in a baking dish.
- Refrigerate the lamb marinade for 4 hours.
- Meanwhile, in a skillet, heat oil and butter then add garlic and rosemary; cook for a minute.
- Once set, add soft bread crumbs, cranberries, pepper and cranberries in the skillet and mix well.
- After 4 hours, remove the baking dish from the refrigerator; serve the marinade juice in a bowl.
- Pat the lamb with the bread crumb mixture and line it on a roasting pan.
- Bake the lamb in the oven for about 30 minutes with a foil on top to prevent burning.
- Once done, allow to cool for 15 minutes before serving.

#38 Spicy Meatballs with Cilantro and Parsley

Meatball ingredients
        1 egg
1 lb. ground beef
1 small finely chopped onion
1/4 tsp. cayenne pepper
1/2 tsp. pepper
2 tbsp. fresh cilantro (minced)
1 tbsp. paprika
3 tbsp. fresh parsley (minced)
2 tbsp. ground cumin
1/4 tsp. ground ginger
1/2 tsp.cinnamon

Ingredients for the Sauce
1 cup of beef broth (organic)
2 tbsp. olive oil
2 cups crushed organic tomatoes
2 medium chopped onions
1/2 tsp. black pepper
1/2 cup parsley (freshly chopped)
4 minced garlic cloves
2 tsp. ground cumin
Pinch of cayenne

Directions
- In a large bowl, mix all meatball ingredients and roll them into large balls.
- In a pan, add the meatballs, and oil; cook for 15 minutes until golden brown.
- Prepare a pot to cook the sauce and set heat to medium high.
- Add olive oil, garlic, pepper, onions, parsley, cayenne and cumin.
- Cook for about 10 minutes, then add the cooked meatballs and simmer for 15 minutes.
- Serve the spicy meatballs with sourdough bread on the side.

#39 Mexican-Inspired Cheesy Pumpkin Soup

Ingredients

1 3/4 cup low-sodium vegetable broth
2/3 cup pumpkin purée
1 can diced tomatoes (reserve liquid)
2 cups Nacho-blend cheese (shredded)
1 Jalapeño
1/4 cup light sour cream
1/4 cup all-purpose flour
Croutons (for garnishing)
Parsley (for garnishing)

Directions

- In a large pot, combine the vegetable broth, pumpkin puree and tomato liquid.
- Cook over medium heat for 3 minutes; remove from heat.
- Stir in nacho-blend cheese, sour cream, jalapeño and tomatoes.
- Cover the pot and bring soup to a boil; serve in individual bowls.
- Garnish with croutons and parsley.
- This recipe serves 2.

#40 Avocado-Ginger and Carrot Soup

Ingredients

1/4 juice of a lemon

1/4 cup Almond Milk

1 tsp. ginger

2 medium carrots (diced)

5 cups water

1 avocado (diced)

Directions

- In a blender, add the lemon, almond milk, ginger, carrots, water and avocado.
- Mix all the ingredients well until a thick cream is achieved.
- Serve the soup cold in a bowl.
- This recipe serves 4.

#41 Creamy Oven-Roasted Onion and Tomato Soup

Ingredients

4 large ripe tomatoes

5 garlic cloves

1/2 medium yellow onion

Ground pepper (to taste)

1 tbsp. olive oil

    1 tbsp. chopped parsley

1 and 1/2 cups almond milk

2 tbsp. tomato paste

Directions

- On a rimmed baking sheet, spread tomatoes and onions.
- Drizzle with the salt, pepper, olive oil, and chopped parsley.
- With your hands, toss the vegetables gently.

- Tuck garlic cloves into the tomato to prevent from burning.
- Oven-roast for 40 minutes at 350 degrees F; remove and cool.
- In a large pot, add the almond milk and tomato paste.
- Add the ingredients into the pot and simmer for about 10 minutes.
- Add water if the creamy soup gets too thick; season with pepper and a little salt to taste.
- Serve immediately and enjoy!

#42 Tomato, Garlic and Bell Pepper Cold Soup

Ingredients

4 tomatoes

1/2 medium white onion

1 clove garlic

Lemon juice to taste

1 cucumber

1 tbsp. virgin olive oil

1 red bell pepper

1 scallion

4 tbsp. freshly chopped cilantro

1/4 cup mango

Directions

- In a blender, add all the ingredients and puree; use a vegetable press to strain the cucumber pits and skin.
- Serve in a bowl and drizzle olive oil, sprinkle chopped scallions, mango and cilantro.
- This recipe serves 4.

#43 Chicken Breast Tomato-Zucchini Salad

Ingredients

2 chicken breasts

2 tbsp. tomato sauce

1/4 cup black olives

1/2 tsp. oregano leaves

½ cup green bell pepper

1 tbsp. unsalted butter

½ cup yellow bell pepper

2 medium zucchini

½ cup red bell pepper

Ground pepper (to taste)

Directions

- Preheat your oven to 250 degrees F.
- In a bowl, add the chicken breast and sprinkle it with ground pepper to taste.
- In a foil wrap, add the zucchini slices and assorted bell peppers.
- Top the vegetable mixture with the chicken, oregano, unsalted butter, tomato sauce and olives.
- Close the foil and bake for 30 minutes; unwrap and serve immediately.

#44 Smoked Turkey with Mango-Arugula Salad

Ingredients
1/4 cup fresh cilantro
1 cup smoked turkey
Lime vinaigrette
4 cups salad greens
2 medium mangoes

Directions
- On a chopping board, peel and slice the ripe mangoes by about 1/8 of an inch.
- Prepare a bowl and add chopped turkey, cilantro; toss in the arugula.
- Serve on a plate and drizzle lime vinaigrette on top.
- The recipe serves 2.

Ingredients for the Lime Vinaigrette
2 tbsp. olive oil
2 tbsp. water
¼ tsp. Lime peel (shredded finely)
1/4 tsp. grated fresh ginger
2 tbsp. lime juice

Directions
- In a glass jar container, mix all the ingredients together, cover the container and vigorously shake to incorporate all the flavors.
- Serve on a small dish as dressing for the salad.

#45 Cranberry Salad in Watercress, Fennel with Balsamic Dressing

Ingredients
2 ounces toasted pecans
225 ml extra virgin olive oil
3 cloves garlic
1 ounce dried cranberries
3 bulbs fennel
3 small heads radicchio

2 tbsp. balsamic vinegar

2 tbsp. red wine vinegar

3 bunches watercress

Directions

- In a small bowl, combine the red wine vinegar, garlic, cranberries, and balsamic vinegar.
- Slowly whisk in the olive oil to emulsify.
- In a large salad bowl, combine the radicchio, watercress, fennel and pecans.
- Pour the balsamic dressing over salad; toss well, top with shavings of non-dairy gorgonzola cheese and serve.

#46 Cheesy Garlic and Basil Pizza

Ingredients

2 tbsp. whole-wheat flour

½ tsp. dried basil

½ cup low-fat ricotta cheese

1 refrigerated whole-wheat pizza crust (store-bought)

2 tbsp. olive oil

4 ounces shredded part-skim mozzarella cheese

2 cups mushrooms

1 large red pepper

1 small onion

2 cloves garlic

Olive oil (for cooking)

Directions

- In a bowl, mix the basil, garlic, onion and ricotta cheese; spread over the piecrust.
- Place the pizza crust onto the cookie sheet, add the red bell pepper, mushrooms and generously sprinkle it with parmesan cheese.
- Bake for about 15 minutes at 425 degrees.

- Remove from the oven and slice the pizza into 8 wedges.
- Serve right away and enjoy!

#47 Turkey with Rosemary and Garlic

Ingredients

3 cloves garlic

2 lb. turkey chunks (thinly sliced)

1/4 cup fresh lemon juice

1 tbsp. black peppercorns

2 tbsp. fresh rosemary

2 tbsp. olive oil

Ground pepper (for seasoning)

Directions

- Preheat your grill and grease the pan with cooking spray.
- In a medium-sized bowl, add the garlic, turkey chunks, lemon juice, peppercorns and rosemary; refrigerate for 1 hour.
- Remove the turkey from marinade and season with ground pepper.
- In a pan, cook the turkey for about 4 minutes; add the remaining lemon juice.
- Serve on a plate and garnish with rosemary leaves.

#48 Chicken Buffalo Crispy Fingers

Ingredients

2 tbsp. apple cider vinegar

2 tsp. garlic powder

2 large eggs

2 tsp. onion powder

2 tsp. paprika

1 juice of a lemon

500 grams chicken tenders

1 cups pork rind oil

Directions

- Preheat oven to 400F.
- Whisk the apple cider vinegar, garlic powder, eggs, onions powder, paprika, and the juice of a lemon in a medium bowl.
- Dip each of the chicken fingers into the egg wash and then lay in the breading together with pork rind oil.
- Place the breaded chicken fingers on a baking sheet and bake for 25 minutes.
- Serve on a plate and enjoy!

#49 Turkey, Bacon and Spinach Scones

Ingredients

12 slices bacon

1 tbsp. bacon fat

6 pieces eggs (whole)

1/2 yellow bell pepper (chopped)

1/2 cup egg whites (liquid)

1 cup spinach (chopped)

¼ cup turkey meat (chopped)

Directions

- In a skillet, fry bacon to a crisp; set aside.
- Preheat the oven to 400 degrees F.
- Line the muffin tins with cooked bacon.
- In the same skillet, retain about 1 tablespoon of bacon fat; scramble the eggs.
- Add the turkey meat, bell pepper and spinach.
- Mix all ingredients and pour into the muffin tins.
- Bake for 30 minutes and store them at room temperature before serving.

- This recipe serves 12. (Note: these miniature muffin/serving consist of 3 pieces)

#50 Tomatoes and Egg Tuna Salad on a Lettuce Roll

Ingredients
1 tbsp. red wine vinegar
1 onion (sliced)
1 can of tuna in olive oil
Black pepper (to taste)
1 juice of a Lemon
5 iceberg lettuce leaves
8 tomato slices
1 hard-boiled egg

Directions
- In a medium-sized bowl, combine the red wine vinegar, onions and lemon juice; set aside for 5 minutes.
- Add the tuna together with its oil and combine with red wine vinegar mixture.
- On a plate, roll the lettuce leaves with tomato slices, tuna salad and sliced eggs.
- This recipe serves 4.

#51 Tuna with Onions, Cabbage and Olives in White Wine Vinegar

Ingredients
1 cabbage (cut into strips)
Ground pepper (to taste)
2 tbsp. white wine vinegar
1/2 cup black olives
1/4 cup of olive oil

1 can of tuna in oil

2 cups fresh curly parsley

1/2 red onion

Directions

- In a salad bowl, add pepper, and white wine vinegar; whisk to emulsify.
- Add the remaining of the ingredients; gently toss to combine.
- Refrigerate for 30 minutes and serve chilled.

#52 Stir-Fry Shrimp with Radish and Snow Peas

Ingredients

20g radish

2 cups shrimp

2/3 teaspoon olive oil

30g snow peas

100ml water

1 tbsp. rice wine

½ tsp. pepper

Directions

- In a medium-sized bowl, soak the radish in water for about 5 minutes; transfer to a pan but reserve its liquid.
- In a pan, stir-fry the shrimp with olive oil; add the snow peas, water, rice wine and pepper.
- Pour the reserve radish liquid to the pan and simmer.
- Serve the shrimps and vegetables on a plate and enjoy!
- This recipe serves 4.

#53 Salmon with Parsnips, Broccoli and Dill

Ingredients

5 ounces salmon (sliced)
1 tbsp. lemon juice
1 tsp. dill
2/3 cup parsnips
1 1/2 cup steamed broccoli

Directions

- Preheat your oven to 225 degrees F.
- In a baking dish, layer on the salmon slices, add lemon juice and sprinkle a teaspoon of dill.
- Bake for about 15 minutes and remove from the oven once the salmon turns flaky.
- Serve on a plate and add the steamed parsnip and broccoli on the side.
- This recipe serves 3.

#54 Maple-Cured Cauliflower Steak with Almond Slivers

Ingredients

1 tbsp. lemon juice

1 tbsp. light maple syrup

1 tbsp. fresh dill

1 tsp. onion powder

1 tbsp. olive oil

¼ cup almonds

1 tsp. basil

1 small head cauliflower

¼ cup red onion

½ tsp. paprika

1 apple

Directions

- On a chopping board, slice the cauliflower and cut into halves.
- Cut the large cauliflower steaks; refrigerate.
- In a food processor, add all the liquid ingredients, chopped apples, maple syrup, olive oil and lemon juice; puree to a sauce-like consistency.
- Add the rest of the ingredients except the almonds and cauliflowers and puree in the food processor.
- In a bowl, transfer the pureed mixture, top with cauliflower slices; sprinkle sliced almonds.
- Dehydrate the mixture for 4 hours and serve on top of the cauliflower steaks.
- This recipe serves 4.

#55 Garlicky Ricotta Bacon and Baby Peppers

Ingredients

6 ounces soft goat cheese

1 tsp. garlic powder

10 sweet mini peppers
10 bacon strips
1/2 cup ricotta cheese
Pepper (to taste)

Directions
- Set oven to broil and line a baking sheet with foil; set aside.
- In a medium-size bowl, add the goat cheese, seasonings, and ricotta.
- Insert the cheese mix in each of the halved peppers; wrap them with bacon.
- Broil the peppers for 12 minutes until light brown; serve.

#56 Sautéed Asparagus, Capers and Pinto Beans

Ingredients
1 lb. asparagus
1 tbsp. olive oil
2 garlic cloves
1½ cups frozen corn kernels
1 cup grape tomatoes
3 scallions
1 can of pinto beans
1 tbsp. capers (diced)
¼ tsp. black pepper

Directions
- In a skillet, cook the garlic for about 30 seconds; set aside.
- Add the corn, asparagus and the beans in the same skillet; cook until tender.
- Stir in the capers and the rest of the ingredients.
- Serve on a plate and garnish with extra grape tomatoes.

Chapter 6. Low-Carb Snack Recipes

Note: for the directions, all smoothies are prepared the same way. Unless otherwise stated that ingredients require cooking before being blended. Otherwise, just combine all ingredients in a blender and process until the desired smooth consistency is achieved.

#57 Strawberry-Banana Flax seed Smoothie

Ingredients
2 tbsp. flaxseed meal
1 cup almond milk (unsweetened)
½ piece of banana
5 ice cubes
1 cup strawberries
Raw honey (to taste)

#58 Banana-Carrot Smoothie

Ingredients
½ cup baby carrots
1 cup cold almond milk (unsweetened)
1 banana
½ tsp. vanilla extract
Raw honey (to taste)
2 tbsp. flax seed meal

#59 Cherry-Almond Milk Smoothie

Ingredients
½ cup yogurt

1 cup almond milk (unsweetened)
1 cup frozen cherries
1 tbsp. raw honey
5 ice cubes

#60 Milky Low-Carb Papaya Smoothie

Ingredients
1 tbsp. raw honey
1/3 cup almond milk
2 cups papaya juice
1 small ripe papaya
6 ice cubes

#61 Avocado Smoothie with Yogurt and Green Tea

Ingredients
1/2 cup plain yogurt
Raw honey (to taste)
1 and 1/4 cup unsweetened almond milk
1 tbsp. water
1 tsp. green tea powder
1/2 medium avocado

#62 Berry Cinnamon Smoothie with Spinach and Chia

Ingredients
1 tsp. ground cinnamon
2 cups spinach
1/4 cup soaked chia seed
1/2 cup strawberries
2 tbsp. walnuts (chopped)
1/2 cup blueberries
Cinnamon powder (for garnishing)
2 cups water (for softening the chia seeds)
        1 tbsp. ground flax seed

Directions
- In a small bowl, add hot water and chia seeds; soften for 30 minutes.

#63 Blueberry-Almond Smoothie

Ingredients
2 tbsp. almond milk
1 and 1/2 cups of fresh blueberries
1/2 cup Greek yogurt (fat-free)
1/4 cup almonds (slivers)
2 tsp. raw honey

Cinnamon powder (for garnishing)
1 cup ice cubes

#64 Strawberry-Banana Yogurt Smoothie

Ingredients
1 cup strawberry yogurt (sugar-free)
1 cup crushed ice
1 cup fresh strawberries
1 banana

#65 Orange, Soy Milk and Banana Smoothie

Ingredients
1 banana
1/4 cup wheat germ
1/2 cup orange juice
1 cup fortified soy milk
Ice

#66 Choco-Vanilla Peanut Butter Festive Latte

Ingredients
1 cup milk
2 cups coffee cubes
¼ cup chocolate syrup
2 tbsp. peanut butter
2 tsp. vanilla extract

Directions
- Prepare the coffee cubes at least 3 hours before making the latte.
- Brew strong coffee, once cool, pour into ice trays; freeze.

#67 Apple-Almond Yogurt Smoothie

Ingredients
½ cup low-fat yogurt
1 apple
1 tsp. cinnamon
1 cup almond milk (unsweetened)
5 almonds

#68 Peach-Banana Almond Milk Smoothie

Ingredients
1 tbsp. flax seed
1 grated ginger
1 small banana
¼ tsp. vanilla extract
1 cup peaches
1 cup cold almond milk
1 oz. Aloe Vera

#69 Apple-Avocado Milk Smoothie

Ingredients
1/2 cup of skim milk
2 tbsp. chia seeds
1/2 avocado
1/2 cup of pineapple (fresh)
1/2 apple
1/2 cup of broccoli (fresh)
1/2 cup of spinach (fresh)
1 cup ice

#70 Banapple Vanilla Almond Smoothie

Ingredients
½ cored apple
1 tsp. cinnamon
Stevia (to taste)
5 ice cubes
1 small carton of vanilla almond milk (unsweetened)
½ piece of banana

#71Vanilla-Apricot Smoothie

Ingredients
1 tbsp. agave syrup
10 apricot halves (dried)
5 ice cubes
1 cup vanilla almond milk (unsweetened)
½ cup yogurt (fat-free)

#72 Strawberry-Banana Flax seed Smoothie

Ingredients
2 tbsp. flaxseed meal
1 cup almond milk (unsweetened)

½ piece of banana
5 ice cubes
1 cup strawberries
Stevia (to taste)

#73 Banana-Carrot Smoothie

Ingredients
½ cup baby carrots
1 cup cold almond milk (unsweetened)
1 frozen banana
½ tsp. vanilla extract
Stevia (sugar substitute to taste)
2 tbsp. flax seed meal

#74 Cherry-Chocolate Milk Smoothie

Ingredients
½ cup yogurt
1 cup cold chocolate almond milk (unsweetened)
1 cup frozen cherries
1 tbsp. honey
5 ice cubes

#75 Papaya Smoothie in Skim Milk and Honey

Ingredients
1tbsp. raw honey
1/3 cup skim milk
2 cups papaya juice
1 small ripe papaya
6 ice cubes

#76 Avocado Power Yogurt Smoothie with Green Tea

Ingredients
1/2 cup plain yogurt
2 tsp. Stevia sugar substitute
1 and 1/4 cup unsweetened almond milk or skim milk
1 tbsp. hot water
1 tsp. green tea powder
1/2 medium avocado

#77 Kale-Strawberry-Lime Smoothie

Ingredients
2 tsp. grated ginger
1 and 1/2 cups of fresh strawberries
6 large kale leaves

2 tsp. honey
3 tbsp. lime juice
1/2 cup cold water

#78 Bok Choy Power Smoothie with Apples and Citrus

Ingredients

1 apple (cored)

1 orange

A handful bok choy

1/2 lemon

1 cup water

2 ice cubes

#79 Fruity Spinach and Ginger Smoothie

Ingredients

2 medium carrots

1 medium apple

2 large baby spinach

1 tbsp. ginger root (freshly grated)

8 ounces water

#80 Kale-Banana Smoothie with Coconut Flakes

Ingredients

1 cup kale leaves

Stevia (to taste)

1 cup water

5 ice cubes

½ piece of banana

3 tbsp. coconut flakes (unsweetened)

#81 Chocolate Cookies in Soymilk

Ingredients

1 unsalted butter (stick)

¾ cup cane sugar

1 cup soymilk

1 tsp. vanilla extract

1 and ¼ cup flour

1 cup chocolate chips

Directions

- Mix cane sugar and butter with a hand mixer.
- Add one cup of soymilk and a teaspoon of vanilla.
- Stir in the chocolate chips and flour.

- Scoop the chocolate batter on ungreased cookie sheet; bake for 12 minutes at 350 degrees F.
- Cool the cookies on a rack before serving.

#82 Cinnamon Bar with Almonds and Apples

Ingredients

3 eggs

1 cup almond meal

1 cored and diced apple

3 tbsp. coconut flour

1 tbsp. cinnamon powder

1/4 cup coconut oil

1 tbsp. raw honey

1/2 tsp. baking soda

Directions

- In a large bowl, whisk eggs, and add coconut oil, coconut flour, almonds, baking soda substitute, and cinnamon powder; mix ingredients until batter is formed.
- On a parchment paper-lined baking tray, scoop small balls and flatten with a fork to make bars.
- Transfer to the oven and bake for 30 minutes at 175 degrees F.
- Once the cinnamon bars are done, cool at room temperature before serving.

#83 Creamy Fruit Salad with Pecan Slivers

Ingredients

1 box instant vanilla pudding mix (sugar-free)

2 cups strawberries

1 can of pineapple tidbits

2 cups grapes

1 lemon juice

1/2 cup water

2 medium apples

2 medium bananas

1/4 cup pecans

Directions

- In a large bowl, add the juice of one lemon, sliced bananas and chopped apples.
- Gently toss the fruit mixture, add the pecans, sliced strawberries, pineapple tidbits and halved grapes; set aside.
- Meanwhile, get another bowl to prepare the creamy mixture.
- Combine water, pineapple juice and the instant pudding mix.
- Use a wired whisk and mix until cream becomes smooth.
- Remove the fruits from the refrigerator and pour the cream mixture on top.
- Gently toss the fruit salad, refrigerate for 30 minutes then serve.

#84 Berry Nutty Fruit Salad

½ can of pineapples tidbits
½ pint blueberries
2 tbsp. instant vanilla pudding mix
½ pint raspberries
1 bunch grapes
1 pound of strawberries

Directions

- In a medium-sized bowl, add the vanilla pudding mix and juice from the fruit cocktail.
- Coat the fruits with the vanilla pudding mixture and refrigerate for about 6 hours.
- Once the fruit cocktail is chilled, remove the bowl from the refrigerator and serve immediately with chopped mixed berries on top.

#85 Light Pistachio-Orange Fruit Salad

Ingredients
1 container frozen whipped topping

1 can of fruit cocktail

2 cups miniature marshmallows

2 large bananas

1 can of pineapple tidbits with juice

1 can of mandarin oranges

1 package pistachio pudding mix

Directions

- In a medium-sized mixing bowl, add the instant pudding mix together with the pineapple tidbits and its juice.
- Mix the whipped topping, marshmallows, bananas, fruit cocktail and oranges.
- Cover the bowl and refrigerate for 3 hours before serving.

#86 Fruit Cocktail Cake with Butter Icing

Ingredients

5 cups fruit cocktail juice

2 eggs

2 tsp. baking soda

2 cups flour

1 and 1/2 cups granulated sugar

Ingredients for the Icing

1 tsp. vanilla

1/2 cup milk

3/4 cup sugar cane

1/2 cup butter

Directions

- Line a medium-sized baking pan with parchment paper.
- In a mixing bowl, mix the sugar, flour, all the contents of the fruit cocktail, cocktail juice, and baking soda.

- Mix all the ingredients until a batter is formed, pour into the greased pans.
- Bake the pans in the oven for about 35 minutes at 350 degrees F.
- Meanwhile, prepare the cake icing by combine vanilla, butter and milk in a saucepan.
- Bring the 4 ingredients to a gentle boil then once it is done, pour over the cake.

#87 Mandarin Oranges and Pineapple Cake

Ingredients
1 package instant vanilla pudding mix
1 package frozen whipped topping
1 can of mandarin oranges
1 package yellow cake mix
1 can crushed pineapple (unsweetened)

Directions
- Preheat your oven to 350 degrees F.
- In two round pans, line them with parchment paper and set aside.
- In a medium-sized bowl, add one package instant vanilla pudding mix with pineapples, eggs and water; mix until smooth.
- Add all the oranges from the can; fold in the pudding mix batter.
- Divide the batter and pour into the lined round pans; bake in the oven for 30 minutes.
- Once the cakes are done, remove them from the pans and transfer to wire racks to cool down.
- Spread the whipped toppings on over the cakes and refrigerate for 30 minutes.

#88 Strawberry with Almond-Vanilla Cream

Ingredients

1 cup almond milk

3 large eggs

1/2 tsp. vanilla extract

1 cup strawberries, pureed

Directions

- Simmer the almond milk in a pot; add vanilla extract and remove from heat.
- In separate bowls, add egg yolks and egg white; beat separately until frothy.
- Add the hot almond milk and vanilla extract to the tempered eggs; freeze for 2 hours.
- In a food processor, puree the sliced strawberries; add the milk mixture, serve in a tall glass to enjoy.

#89 Bacon and Broccoli Egg Rollers

Ingredients

1 small bunch of spinach

¼ cup sliced and diced mushrooms

6 strips of cooked bacon

1/2 cup broccoli

12 eggs

Cooking spray (vegetable oil)

1 small bell pepper

Raw honey (for topping)

Directions

- Heat the oven at 350 degrees F.
- Line muffin tins with cooking spray.
- In a skillet, add the bacon strips and cook it to a crisp.
- Once the bacon is done, chop into little pieces.
- Break 12 eggs and mix with the broccoli, pepper, bacon, spinach and mushrooms.

- In a colander, rinse and drain the broccoli before cutting it into little pieces.
- Pour the egg mix into the muffin tin and bake in the oven for about 25 minutes.
- When cooked, garnish with a few bacon slices and raw honey.

#90 Cinnamon-Vanilla Pumpkin Cuppycakes

Ingredients
1 tsp. cinnamon
15 oz. canned pumpkin
½ spice cake mix
1 tsp. vanilla extract
1 cup water

Directions
- Preheat your oven to 350 degrees F and line a cupcake pan with cupcake paper sleeves.
- In a bowl, mix all five ingredients and slowly pour the batter into the cupcake sleeves.
- Bake for 25 minutes until the cupcakes turn lightly brown and moist.
- Allow the cakes to cool for a bit before removing them from the pan.
- Serve on a plate and enjoy!

Conclusion

Thank you again for purchasing this book!

CHECK OUT MY BOOK ON PALEO DIET: " <u>A Beginner's Guide</u> <u>to the Paleo Diet: A Simple Start to Achieving Optimal Health</u> <u>and Weight Loss through the Original Human Diet + 35 FREE</u> <u>RECIPES"</u>

I hope this book was able to help you understand the benefits of starting a low carb diet. It is indeed one of the healthy alternatives you need to incorporate in your meals. In the previous chapters, you were given a walk-through on the benefits of maintaining a low carb diet. Consider this diet as a long-term choice in order to keep your weight in check while eating the food you love.

The 90 different low carbohydrate recipes provided have flavor variations. 90% of the time, dieters find it boring to keep on eating the same food. This is your chance to whip up mouthwatering meals that still have the same low-carb content you need.

Start preparing meals that will benefit you and your family's health. Isn't it amazing to be given a chance to plot different meals you can mix and match at any given day?

Visit www.projectkt.com for more books!

Finally,

Leave a review for this book on Amazon!

Thank you and good luck!

www.ingramcontent.com/pod-product-compliance
Lightning Source LLC
Chambersburg PA
CBHW071226280526
45787CB00002B/819